For the Girls

by **D. Avery**

EXETER PRESS : NANTUCKET

1st edition - Exeter Press

ISBN: 978-1-365-02221-0

Karen

The Girls

The girls. Ta-tas. Boobs. Knockers. All the rest.
Breasts.
We learn to live with them.

Unless.
Some of us have to get them off our chests.
And learn living without them.

Except.
Some, dear friends, couldn't live.
With or without them.

We live yet.
Learning.
And all the rest.

Knockers

Not perky; ponderous.
Ponderous pendulums swing
from my chest. Knock, knock.
Tick, tock, ticking time. Chimes
of women. When's mine?
My time (knock, knock) of weightiness
of waiting on the radiologist?
Time is a waiting room, the space before
unveiled doom.

Eyes up here!
It's where I'll do my best;
Brave face, forget the breasts.
Or, just knock them off, why wait?
Lift the ponderous weight from off my chest.
Tick, tock.
Time
a wondering heaviness.
Malignant?
Benign?
Knock, knock.

Landings

Since the call-back
There's a split, two kinds of time.
Well, there's before and after of course,
And there's the landings, and the space between.

Landings; each procedure, consult, report, treatment.
Here you catch your breath
here you get your bearings.
Landings are the time when you get information.
Here they tell you something, do something.
And send you on.

The space between landings; here you swim in what-ifs;
Here you tread murky unknowns, uncertainties.
This is an arduous waiting.
A time when questions circle ever closer.
Here you just keep your head up and mark the next
landing.

In between you continue
As if time had not split.
Adrift, easier than answering questions
Of remembering or not remembering
The deep breaths taken at the landings.
And at each successive landing
You seek the ineluctable shore.

Name Games

There is a reciprocal power in naming, beware.
It shows the power of the namer as it bestows
power to the named, so speak with care.

I

The first group of namers was from Pathology,
They bluntly named what they had looked to see,
Pathologists come across as hacks,
Their naming is hardly exact
But names create reality
And though they didn't have many answers,
They loosed fear with one word: cancer.

II

The next group of doctors was more precise
Words as tools, wielded as knife
Their words had power to contain and defuse
Their words carved the best out of bad news
They spoke more accurately, with more precision
Used naming to know, to inform decisions
They had more words, they had more answers
These were the ones who would excise the cancer.

III

Here's the thing about naming
There's reciprocation, a claiming
So don't use possessive pronouns, don't call this thing
"mine"
Don't give it attention, don't give it time.
Don't be named either, don't be Brave, or Scared, or
Tough.
Don't be A Fighter, though fight you must.
Don't use names that show pride
Provocations incite it to thrive.
It thrives on challenge, it thrives on attention;
do not deny, but also don't mention
it; you are not its host, it's not a guest
it is uninvited, unwelcome, and it is time that it left.
Let the namers use their words and weapons
But don't you claim it, show no acception.

IV

So bring on the surgeons, the radiologists
Do as they say, they are experts in this
They know of which they speak
Let them mend the breach
and recreate your former reality
when they speak the words: cancer free.

Intrusion

A proper home invasion is sudden, violent, abrupt
A smashed window, a kicked in door in the night
You get to use your adrenaline rush
You see the intruder, you have something to fight.

There's another intruder who lacks
Even the decency of mice or rats
that at least show themselves at night
To show they've been in the house all along,
only sometimes out of sight.

Why would you suspect your own house?
Relax, there's nothing, or maybe only a mouse.
Why would you suspect there's something there
Quiet as anxiety, maybe under the stairs
Or up in the attic, just biding its time
A squatter in the house you blithely call "mine"?

You wouldn't suspect
though you might make the rounds
Because sometimes you imagine
that you have heard sounds
But you find nothing, must be the house
giving voice to its years
Just an aging house, still pretty solid
you've nothing to fear.

Except the fear that maybe you've overlooked
a silent intruder who lurks in some nook
and lacks the grace to be obvious and abrupt
who instead lingers and waits to erupt
from within not without, insidious violation;
how will you extricate this invisible insinuation?

Christmas Present

Three weeks before Christmas
Santa's working on stuffing his sack.
I make a second appointment
I got a call back.
Radiology wants to squeeze me some more
another look, just to be sure.
Calcifications! Something new that I learned
They said there was a chance that these were of concern.

So a week before Christmas
I'm on a Farmer Frankenstein table
and am told to lie as still as I'm able.
They'd asked many questions, about hormones and
discharge and am I still menstrual
then prodded and poked my boob
with a needle as thick as a pencil.
I headed for home, left boob slightly bruised
anxiously waiting for their biopsy news.
My Christmas promise was that they'd give me an answer
two days before Christmas, surprise! It is cancer.

While visions of iphones dance in young children's heads
I dash away fear, I dash away dread.
For this is the easy one, it occurs very often
but they'll tell me more if I can get up to Boston.

Three days after Christmas,
I meet the team at Mass General
to decide on a plan to keep me non-ephemeral
like my grandmother who may have given a gift;
the results of the gene test may make the plan shift.

But as it is now, in Christmas present,
a lumpectomy is planned, to get this thing out
followed by radiation to remove any doubt.
So while others are crashing from Christmas hype
and anticipation just past
my time of awaiting just seems to last.
Now I await more results
and more decisions to start the new year
But what can I say?
It's good to be here.

Get Well Cards

Have you noticed
The power of words?
It starts with *suspicious,* an implied, possible threat
You're left to imagine, but you know nothing yet.
And after the *c* word is used by pathology
It still takes a while to say it is the best that it could be;
It being it.
They still want to get rid of it.
Okay.

Have you noticed
That even after beginning
With "There are no words"
Or "I don't know what to say"
That speaker keeps speaking anyway?
Here come the clichés,
The tired phrases that really don't fit;
Others' words will always be inadequate.
Whatever; I'm fine.

Have you noticed
That people are "sorry"? What did they do?
Oh- it seems they are sorry for you.
They mean well, they compliment you, say "How tough",
And, "How brave", but they fear that you aren't scared
enough.
Condolences and sympathies;
Some have started the eulogy.
I wish they wouldn't.

There is a group that really shouldn't.
You make an appointment for a procedure
And they say "so sorry that you need to be here"
These are the professionals, who administer
and interpret the tests
But then they wish you good luck,
say they hope for the best
I guess what they're implying about doctors and science
Is that you might rely on another Alliance.

I'll take the science
and the Alliance
I'll do the best that I can.
I imagine that all mean well
And well I imagine I am.

Dream Change

take charge
make change
don't let worry
become sorry
no sorrow
the morrow
always dawns
spawns hope
doors to open
pull, pry
push, try

so be scared
then pick scared up
and mold it
shape it and rearrange
but don't forever hold it
create peace
a place
to keep
your cares
hold sacred
something you can learn from

always be a dreamer
in dreaming be remade
love, live
life, lift
gift, give
live, love
dream
a sacred change
in dreaming
be remade

Until the End

What if, what if?
What if your friend said jump off a cliff?
Is that something that you would do
if it were an experience your friend went through?

What do you truly think is worse;
to be the second, or to be the first?
(Of course there was no cliff jump dare
Just two people with lives to bear)

Even two who call each other friend,
One cannot follow another to her end
But one can be there until the last
Hold her hand but let her pass.

Left alone at the edge of the abyss
Hearing the echoes of all the what ifs
Would you rather be
the one who leads or the one who has to see?

You never ever can be too sure
of all that you truly can endure.
But when there's something to overcome
then you might just be the one.

Neither friend was spared in this
Yet one is left to gather up the lessons
and count them as a gift.

Then

Oh my friend, even the snow didn't
know if it was coming or going never
alighting drifting down floating
up swirling and dancing outside
your fifth floor window overlooking
glistening trees sequined with ice.
And it was spring, by rights; April
and a winter with no end, friend.
So slowly it went
went in a tired melting
grey and gristly snow heaps shrinking
at their edges their strength seeping away.
I saw a lone crocus, yellow
beaming with the hope of spring then
I knew
I knew you were at peace.

Now

Now I see you
sometimes in dreams.
The last time, you were a tree
or were trapped in a tree,
that was trapped in a pot.
A stunted, potted balsam fir you were
in that dream.

I wish I'd slept longer.
To be with you was good
to free you would have been better.
I wish that you could
have told me
what to do.
Before awaking I had thought
to bring you to Vermont
maybe plant you there.
Now I think you needed more
more than transplanting
in that dream.

No, if I could sleep on this
I'd not commit you
to any geography, nor to the time
it takes to be a tree.
You wanted to be free;
your breath caught on every needle;
cellular rooms you wandered
through root and stem
incessantly.

I wish I'd slept longer.
I should pull you from that pot
I would give up selfish thoughts;
No transplanting;
Transformation!
I'd release you through fire.

Oh, how balsam crackles and sparks!
Brightly, briefly flashes
vibrant stars then ashen
flutters dark.
And how it breaks my heart
that I awakened too early from that dream
when you appeared to me
as a tree.

The Radiation Ward

Not mere magazines here;
These waiting rooms have chapter books on shelves
And puzzles.

The whole place is a puzzle
A labyrinth, layered
Without to within.

With-out: reception, exam rooms, outer waiting room
With-in: doctors' offices, changing room, inner waiting
room
At the center: technicians, radiation machine, and Us.

For Each of Us our days are puzzle pieces
Tumbled about and scattered, We have to
Daily find the edges, the corners, build on from here.

We in the inner waiting room
We talk and We joke together as only We can;
We do not work on the puzzle that is on the table.

We have Each been the puzzle on the table
Each different, but for Each the solution now
Is here with the shared machines, the shared technicians.

Our shared puzzle picture here is a shifting kaleidoscope
One of Us will finish,
Someone else will come in, a Beginner.

One by one Each of Us will leave the labyrinth
Find the way back to our own Before
To make a picture whole
a private picture that has had a missing piece.

Jeannie's Radiation Graduation *3/8/16*

Jeannie, not in a bottle
Jeannie not in your dreams
Jeannie some kind of model
Jeannie is more than she seems.

Maybe this isn't funny
But I just couldn't resist;
Her boobs are relocated tummy
Her nipples, well they don't exist.

But she's always wanted a tattoo
And a boob job to get the girls down to size
Oh the things that some people go through
A nightmare for dreams realized.

Bald brought out her eyes of blue
When chemo took out her hair
She said, "Cancer, fuck you"
She never appeared to be scared.

She's my fearless leader
Older and more experienced
I wish I didn't need her
For her cancer sense.

But she has boldly gone
And now she's finally done;
Happy graduation
Now go forth, have fun.

March 8; International Women's Day

Some women.
Some women had their last treatment today
Some their first
Some were untreated.

Some had heart attacks, some died
Some lived.
Some women felt dead inside
Others felt vibrant and alive.

Baby girls were born today
borne of women become mothers
While others became aunts, mentors, friends.
Today, and yesterday, and tomorrow
Some will feel joy, some will feel sorrow.

Some women were betrayed today
Some endured violence and pain
Fell down, got pushed around
Got up, tried again.

Women endured today.
Some were supported, some were supportive
Some felt hate, some were hated
Some gave love, some were loved.

Around the world, women endure
Some fall ill, some rise cured
Some are able to feel the hope and the good
Of a worldwide sisterhood.

Susan's poem 3/17/16

It's been a journey, you've traveled far
Now you've circled back and know who you are.
Stupid is forever, cancer is not
It helps you be grateful for all that you've got.

You are still standing, you have stood down dread
And you are not stupid, and you are not dead.
From your fair country the snakes have been driven
Now go on, and enjoy lots of living.

So thank you Saint Patrick and Mother Mary too
And I thank you Susan, for just being you.
You've graduated, I'll miss you, that's my sweet sorrow
And I wonder who you'll bare for, come this time to-
morrow.

Tom's poem 3/18/16

No more daily radiant zap zap zaps
You'll need new excuses to excuse your snooze naps
No more mornings with the girls
Get on back to your former world
Good luck with whatever you may do
This part is over, congrats, Tom, you're through.

Graduation Thank You CCH

I'm another gal from Nantucket
Who into your ward was inducted
I got thirty days
To receive your warm rays
Another delay to kicking the bucket.

I certainly didn't plan this
Traveling daily to Hyannis
Who knew radiation
Would become my vacation
And I would revel in such grandness?

For thirty mornings a queen
I dress for spa, for tanning machine
A few moments of respite and rest
Result, one very tan breast
I've basked in the relaxing routine.

March, hate month on the island
But here everybody was smiling
Here there's no hate
You all are great
You are a staff to rely on.

Always professional and efficient
Mere humans now seem deficient
What can compare
To such wonderful care?
In a word you're truly magnificent.

My Commencement   *4/1/16*

I caught a bit of cancer, truly, just a touch
I had it just a little, but it has given me so much.

Now it's my turn to be finished, it's my graduation
End of an era of treatment, no more radiation

A friend said "Hey that's great, now put it in the past"
But I have to say, "I hope the good parts always last."

And maybe this experience has bordered on obsession
But I've learned so much, garnered so many lessons.

It was personal enough last spring when I saw my dear
friend die
Her body scarred and torn, her Self still peering from
tired eyes.

My neighbor diagnosed, through her I shed more
ignorance
About what so many women go through, for me another
third person experience.

That should have been enough; I showed support and
empathy
But the next lesson was a diagnosis, a diagnosis this time
for me.

I learned first hand of waiting
Time when worry tries to have its way
The flip side is appreciation
Appreciation for each God given day

Maybe these are asides, fodder for a different poem,
It's my graduation, I really do want to get going.
So thank you everybody, for your kindness and your care
But my thirty days are done, now I'm out of here.

I'm In Charge of Celebrations *4/1/16*

Friend, you were here, the day I celebrated.
You kept wishing for sunshine
and it was a rainy, foggy day
but friend, the sun was shining.

Some days when I flew, it would be grey and drizzly
and then we'd climb and be in dazzling sunshine
above the endless white cloud plains.
I'd laugh then, and think about perspective
even as we descended, returning to a rainy day.
Because, friend, the sun was shining.

Some days it was cold, the wind whipping me along
and people would say, why didn't you call me for a
ride?
A ride? If I didn't walk I'd just have more time to
wait, inside.
Outside the birds were singing up the day, bringing
spring with their song. A ride? No.
The birds warmed me on my walk
and friend, the sun was shining.

Some days I met people who had nothing,
nothing but stories
and all they wanted was for someone to listen,
so I did.
And I met people who had lots but they
wasted time and brought stress
by complaining and being impatient.
So when there were delays I learned patience
and listened for a story.
Friend, I got where I needed to go,
and the sun shone.

Some days I was tired, so I allowed myself to do less.
I listened to my body and I let others help me
and you were one of those helpers, friend.
That same sun that is sometimes hidden from view,
that same moon that is sometimes shrouded in
cloud, do you see them too friend?
Greatly I have traveled, and never did I travel alone.

Though the garden blooms
she wearies in her body
flowers go unpicked.

Gone before autumn harvest
gone with winter's winds;
Only birds returned this spring.

When

"It's not if, but when"
an observation of a friend.
And we might
be left
to wonder
if not when,
then who?
Who next?
So many someones
someone's loved one
who is next
who is right now
being asked
and ask themselves
how?
How bad? How long?
And we ask how they are
always "hopeful", always "strong"
and we wonder
and they must too,
ask, if not why,
then when?
When is it enough?

Aftermath

there's the aftermath and the math that came before
the math beginning
at conception
studies in symmetry
cell division
beyond your perception
dividing dividing
doubling doubling
whole greater than the sum of its parts

that math was before
now you are older and there is more
increase of everything
increase of years
increase of knowledge of what you might fear

there's simple math, the hardest math
more than two hands can handle
simply counting those we know
diagnosed
fractions and subtractions
impossible math of infinite cost
enumerating
those we have lost

and maybe you become
one that's counted
diagnosed
now doing the math of probability
careful computation of likelihood
of outcomes
positive or negative
percentages and rates
varying possibilities
including remission
including recurrence
check the math
compute for assurance
the math meant to be descriptive
expressions of comparative measures
of stages and of grades
the math of measures
of counting time
of duration
days of radiation
rounds of chemo
years of expectation

weighing quantity and quality
calculating how long
this kind of math is wrong.

These Ones

Survivors are ones
who live without their loved one
They're the ones who mourn.

Here's a survivor;
who will taste the soup he makes
at the stove alone?
Heavily he stirs
spices that she never liked
says now it doesn't matter
stirs in even more
for this is what matters most.
At the stove he mourns.

Another, a girl
gathering ingredients
on her twelfth birthday
another year passed.
Alone at her mother's stove
she bakes her own cake.

Others, grown children
cry still for understanding
struggle to forgive
burdened with too much
weakened by their loss
in their own kitchens mourning.

In them all see hope
with each meal that they prepare
with each bite they take.

Favored recipes
revisions and additions;
Bitter sweet their task.

That Girl

do you keep in touch with her?
you know, that girl that you once were?

I think you should
I hope you do
remember her
she remembers you

she doesn't need to be forgiven
doesn't need to forgive you
she just wonders how you're doing
she hasn't forgotten you

she'd like it if where you're going
you would bring her along
she wants to help you get there
she'll help you to be strong

don't forget her
try to make some time
know that you
have always been on her mind

Letting go...
Where am I?
Here I am.
I am.
I?
?
.

Thy.
Thy will.
Thy will be.
Thy will be done.
Letting go, letting God

Letting go, letting God
Thy will be done
Thy will be
Thy will
Thy
I
I am
I am here
Here I am...
Letting go, letting God
...

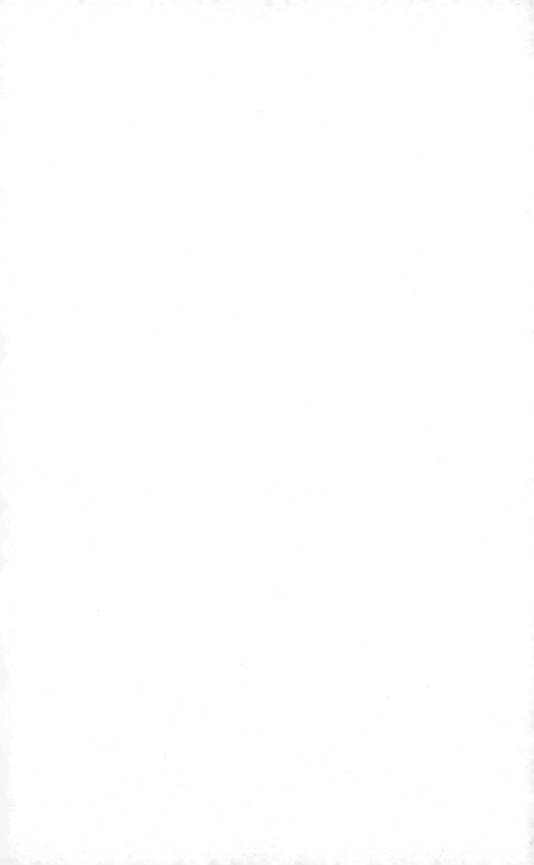

72709604R00038

Made in the USA
Columbia, SC
23 June 2017